BUDGET-FRIENDLY DIABETIC COOKBOOK FOR THE NEWLY DIAGNOSED

2000+ Days of wallet-friendly delicious diabetic diet recipes for pre-diabetes, type 2 diabetes and newly diagnosed, with a 31day meal plan

Nathan Wendy

Table of Contents

COPYRIGHT © 2023

CHAPTER ONE

Introduction to Diabetes and Budget-Friendly Cooking

Diabetes is a chronic condition characterized by high levels of sugar (glucose) in the blood. It occurs when the body either does not produce enough insulin (a hormone that regulates blood sugar) or cannot effectively use the insulin it produces. This leads to elevated blood sugar levels, which can cause a range of health complications if not properly managed. Budget-friendly cooking, on the other hand, involves preparing nutritious meals while minimizing costs. For individuals with diabetes, managing both their condition and their budget can be challenging, but with the right knowledge and strategies, it is possible to eat healthily without breaking the bank.

Understanding Diabetes: A Beginner's Guide

Diabetes is classified into several types, with the most common being type 1, type 2, and gestational diabetes. Type 1 diabetes typically develops during childhood or adolescence and occurs when the immune system attacks and destroys the insulin-producing cells in the pancreas. People with type 1 diabetes require insulin injections to survive. Type 2 diabetes is more common and often develops in adulthood, although it is increasingly being diagnosed in children and adolescents due to rising obesity rates. In type 2 diabetes, the body becomes resistant to insulin or does not produce enough insulin to meet its needs. Gestational diabetes occurs during pregnancy and usually resolves after childbirth, but it increases the risk of developing type 2 diabetes later in life.

Managing diabetes involves maintaining blood sugar levels within a target range through a combination of medication, diet, exercise, and regular monitoring. Monitoring blood sugar levels allows individuals to adjust their treatment regimen as needed to prevent complications such as heart disease, stroke, kidney failure, and nerve damage.

Importance of Budget-Friendly Cooking for Diabetes Management

Eating a healthy diet is essential for managing diabetes and reducing the risk of complications. However, many people believe that eating healthily means spending more money on groceries, which can be a barrier for those on a tight budget. Budget-friendly cooking for diabetes management is important because it allows individuals to prioritize their health without overspending. By making smart food choices and using cost-saving strategies, such as buying in bulk, shopping for seasonal produce, and minimizing food waste, it is possible to create nutritious meals that are both affordable and delicious.

Budget-friendly cooking can also help individuals with diabetes maintain a healthy weight, which is important for managing blood sugar levels and reducing the risk of complications. By focusing on whole foods such as fruits, vegetables, lean proteins, and whole grains, and minimizing the consumption of processed and high-calorie foods, it is possible to achieve better blood sugar control and overall health without breaking the bank.

Tips for Eating Healthy on a Budget

1. **Plan Ahead:** Planning meals in advance can help individuals with diabetes make healthier choices and avoid impulse purchases. Take inventory of pantry staples and plan meals around ingredients that are already on hand. Create a weekly meal plan and shopping list based on budget-friendly recipes and seasonal produce.

2. **Buy in Bulk:** Purchasing staple items such as rice, beans, pasta, and oats in bulk can help save money in the long run. Look for sales and discounts on non-perishable items and consider joining a wholesale club or co-op to access lower prices on bulk items.

3. **Shop for Seasonal Produce:** Seasonal fruits and vegetables are often more affordable and better quality than out-of-season produce. Visit farmers' markets or local produce stands to find fresh, seasonal produce at lower prices. Consider buying extra and freezing or preserving fruits and vegetables to enjoy them throughout the year.

4. **Focus on Plant-Based Proteins:** Plant-based proteins such as beans, lentils, tofu, and tempeh are typically less expensive than animal proteins and can be just as nutritious. Incorporate meatless meals into your weekly meal plan to save money and improve your health.

5. **Minimize Food Waste:** According to the Food and Agriculture Organization of the United Nations, approximately one-third of all food produced for human consumption is lost or wasted each year. Minimizing food waste can help individuals save money and reduce their environmental impact. Plan meals based on perishable items that need to be used up and store leftovers properly to extend their shelf life.

6. **Cook at Home:** Eating out can be expensive and often involves larger portion sizes and higher calorie foods. Cooking at home allows individuals to control portion sizes, ingredients, and cooking methods, making it easier to stick to a healthy eating plan. Experiment with budget-friendly recipes and cooking techniques to create nutritious meals that are both affordable and satisfying.

7. **Use Coupons and Discounts:** Take advantage of coupons, sales, and discounts to save money on groceries. Sign up for loyalty programs at your favorite grocery stores and look for digital coupons and discount codes online. Consider using

cash-back apps and rebate programs to earn rewards on your grocery purchases.

8. **Limit Processed Foods:** Processed and convenience foods are often more expensive and less nutritious than whole foods. Limiting the consumption of processed foods such as sugary snacks, frozen meals, and pre-packaged snacks can help individuals save money and improve their health. Focus on cooking from scratch using whole ingredients whenever possible.

In conclusion, managing diabetes on a budget requires careful planning, smart shopping, and creative cooking. By prioritizing nutritious foods, minimizing costs, and making the most of available resources, individuals with diabetes can eat healthily without overspending. With the right strategies and support, it is possible to achieve better blood sugar control, improve overall health, and enjoy delicious meals that won't break the bank.

CHAPTER TWO

Planning Budget-Friendly Diabetic Meals

Meal planning is a crucial aspect of managing diabetes on a budget. It involves carefully selecting nutritious foods, creating balanced meals, and minimizing costs. By planning ahead and utilizing cost-saving strategies, individuals with diabetes can eat healthily without overspending. This chapter will explore the basics of meal planning for diabetes on a budget, smart shopping tips to save money on groceries, and techniques for stretching ingredients and making the most of leftovers.

Basics of Meal Planning for Diabetes on a Budget

Meal planning for diabetes involves creating balanced meals that help manage blood sugar levels while also being affordable. The key principles of meal planning for diabetes include:

1. **Balanced Plate:** Aim to include a variety of foods from different food groups in each meal to ensure a balanced intake of nutrients. Fill half of your plate with non-starchy vegetables such as leafy greens, broccoli, and bell peppers, one-quarter with lean proteins such as chicken, fish, tofu, or beans, and one-quarter with whole grains or starchy vegetables such as brown rice, quinoa, or sweet potatoes.

Add a serving of healthy fats such as olive oil, nuts, or avocado to round out the meal.

2. **Portion Control:** Pay attention to portion sizes to prevent overeating and manage calorie intake. Use measuring cups, spoons, or visual cues to estimate portion sizes and avoid oversized servings. Eating smaller, more frequent meals throughout the day can help regulate blood sugar levels and prevent spikes and crashes.

3. **Carbohydrate Management:** Carbohydrates have the most significant impact on blood sugar levels, so it's essential to monitor carbohydrate intake and choose carbohydrates that have a minimal impact on blood sugar, such as whole grains, legumes, and non-starchy vegetables. Limit refined carbohydrates and sugary foods, which can cause blood sugar spikes.

4. **Meal Timing:** Spread carbohydrate intake evenly throughout the day and aim for consistency in meal timing to help regulate blood sugar levels. Avoid skipping meals or going long periods without eating, as this can lead to fluctuations in blood sugar levels.

5. **Variety and Flexibility:** Keep meals interesting by incorporating a variety of flavors, textures, and cuisines. Experiment with different recipes and ingredients to prevent boredom and ensure adequate nutrient intake. Be flexible

with meal plans and adapt them based on individual preferences, dietary restrictions, and budget constraints.

Shopping Smart: Budget-Friendly Grocery Tips

Smart shopping is essential for sticking to a budget while purchasing nutritious foods for diabetes management. Consider the following tips to save money on groceries:

1. **Make a Shopping List:** Before heading to the grocery store, make a list of items you need based on your meal plan and pantry inventory. Stick to the list to avoid impulse purchases and reduce the risk of overspending.

2. **Shop the Perimeter:** The perimeter of the grocery store typically contains fresh produce, dairy, meat, and seafood, while the inner aisles contain processed and packaged foods. Focus on shopping the perimeter to prioritize whole, nutrient-dense foods and minimize the temptation to buy unnecessary items.

3. **Compare Prices:** Compare prices between different brands and store options to find the best deals on staple items. Consider purchasing generic or store-brand products, which are often cheaper than name-brand equivalents without sacrificing quality.

4. **Buy in Bulk:** Purchase non-perishable items such as grains, beans, and spices in bulk to save money in the long run. Look

for bulk bins or larger package sizes to take advantage of discounted prices.

5. **Use Coupons and Discounts:** Look for coupons, sales, and discounts on grocery items to save money. Clip coupons from newspapers or online sources, sign up for loyalty programs at your favorite stores, and take advantage of digital coupons and rebate offers.

6. **Shop Seasonally:** Purchase fruits and vegetables that are in season to take advantage of lower prices and better quality produce. Visit farmers' markets or local produce stands to find fresh, seasonal produce at competitive prices.

7. **Avoid Impulse Buys:** Stick to your shopping list and avoid impulse purchases, especially items that are not essential to your meal plan. Avoid shopping when hungry, as this can lead to impulse buys and overspending.

8. **Consider Frozen and Canned Options:** Frozen and canned fruits and vegetables are often more affordable and have a longer shelf life than fresh produce. Stock up on frozen and canned options to have nutritious ingredients on hand for quick and convenient meals.

Stretching Ingredients and Making the Most of Leftovers

Stretching ingredients and making the most of leftovers are essential strategies for maximizing your food budget and reducing waste. Consider the following tips:

1. **Meal Prep:** Spend some time each week prepping ingredients and cooking in bulk to save time and money. Cook large batches of grains, beans, and proteins and portion them out for use in multiple meals throughout the week.

2. **Repurpose Leftovers:** Get creative with leftovers by repurposing them into new meals. For example, leftover roasted vegetables can be added to salads, soups, or omelets, while cooked grains can be used as a base for grain bowls or stir-fries.

3. **Freeze Leftovers:** If you have leftover meals that you won't be able to eat right away, freeze them for later use. Invest in freezer-safe containers or resealable bags and label them with the contents and date for easy identification.

4. **Use Scraps and Peels:** Don't discard vegetable scraps and peels—instead, use them to make homemade broth or stock. Save vegetable scraps such as carrot tops, onion skins,

and celery leaves in a resealable bag in the freezer until you have enough to make broth.

5. **Plan for Repeated Ingredients:** When meal planning, incorporate ingredients that can be used in multiple meals to minimize waste. For example, if you're buying a bunch of cilantro for a recipe, plan to use the remaining cilantro in other dishes throughout the week.

By following these strategies for meal planning, smart shopping, and ingredient stretching, individuals with diabetes can eat healthily on a budget without sacrificing taste or nutrition. With a little planning and creativity, it is possible to enjoy delicious meals while staying within financial constraints.

CHAPTER THREE

Simple and Affordable Breakfasts

Breakfast is often hailed as the most important meal of the day, especially for individuals managing diabetes. A well-balanced breakfast can help stabilize blood sugar levels, provide energy for the day ahead, and kick-start metabolism. However, finding simple and affordable breakfast options that are also diabetes-friendly can be challenging. In this chapter, we will explore budget-friendly breakfast ideas for busy mornings, low-cost options for stable blood sugar, and strategies for breakfast meal prep on a budget.

Budget-Friendly Breakfast Ideas for Busy Mornings

Mornings can be hectic, making it tempting to skip breakfast or opt for convenience foods that may not be the healthiest choice. However, with a little planning and creativity, it's possible to enjoy a nutritious breakfast without breaking the bank. Here are some budget-friendly breakfast ideas for busy mornings:

1. **Overnight Oats:** Overnight oats are a convenient and customizable breakfast option that can be prepared in advance and enjoyed on the go. Simply combine rolled oats with milk or yogurt, add your favorite toppings such as fruit, nuts, and seeds, and let it sit in the refrigerator overnight. In the morning, grab and go for a quick and satisfying breakfast.

2. **Smoothies:** Smoothies are a great way to pack in nutrients and get a quick breakfast fix. Use frozen fruits, leafy greens, protein powder, and liquid of your choice (such as milk, yogurt, or water) to create a balanced and refreshing meal. Make a big batch and pour into individual containers for easy grab-and-go convenience.

3. **Whole Grain Toast:** Toast up some whole grain bread and top it with nut butter, sliced banana, and a sprinkle of cinnamon for a simple and satisfying breakfast. You can also top your toast with avocado, tomato, and a drizzle of olive oil for a savory twist.

4. **Greek Yogurt Parfait:** Layer Greek yogurt with granola and fresh or frozen berries for a protein-packed breakfast that will keep you full until lunchtime. Experiment with different flavors of yogurt and toppings to keep things interesting.

5. **Egg Muffins:** Whip up a batch of egg muffins filled with vegetables, cheese, and lean protein for a portable and protein-rich breakfast option. Make a big batch on the weekend and reheat them throughout the week for a quick and easy breakfast on busy mornings.

6. **Homemade Breakfast Bars:** Skip the store-bought granola bars and make your own at home using oats, nuts, seeds, dried fruit, and a touch of honey or maple syrup for

sweetness. Bake them in a large batch and store them in an airtight container for a convenient breakfast or snack option.

7. **Leftover Breakfast Burritos:** Use leftover cooked vegetables, beans, and protein (such as chicken or tofu) to fill whole grain tortillas for a hearty and portable breakfast option. Wrap them up and freeze them individually for a quick and easy breakfast on busy mornings.

8. **DIY Instant Oatmeal Packets:** Make your own instant oatmeal packets by combining rolled oats, dried fruit, nuts, and spices in individual baggies. When you're ready to eat, simply pour the contents into a bowl, add hot water or milk, and microwave for a quick and easy breakfast.

Low-Cost Breakfast Options for Stable Blood Sugar

For individuals managing diabetes, it's essential to choose breakfast options that help stabilize blood sugar levels and provide sustained energy throughout the morning. Here are some low-cost breakfast options that are gentle on blood sugar:

1. **High-Fiber Cereals:** Look for whole grain cereals that are high in fiber and low in added sugars. Pair your cereal with milk or yogurt and add fresh fruit for extra flavor and nutrients.

2. **Egg-Based Dishes:** Eggs are a budget-friendly source of protein and can be prepared in countless ways. Try scrambled eggs with vegetables, a veggie omelet, or hard-boiled eggs paired with whole grain toast for a balanced breakfast.

3. **Chia Seed Pudding:** Chia seeds are packed with fiber and protein, making them an excellent choice for stabilizing blood sugar levels. Mix chia seeds with milk or yogurt and let them sit in the refrigerator overnight to create a creamy and nutritious pudding. Top with fresh fruit or nuts for added flavor and texture.

4. **Vegetable Frittata:** Whip up a vegetable frittata using leftover vegetables, eggs, and cheese for a hearty and satisfying breakfast that's low in carbs and high in protein. Bake it in a large batch and slice it into individual portions for easy reheating throughout the week.

5. **Cottage Cheese Bowl:** Cottage cheese is a low-cost source of protein that pairs well with a variety of toppings. Mix cottage cheese with fruit, nuts, and a drizzle of honey or maple syrup for a sweet and savory breakfast option.

6. **Homemade Breakfast Sandwiches:** Skip the drive-thru and make your own breakfast sandwiches at home using whole grain English muffins or bagels, eggs, cheese, and lean protein such as turkey sausage or Canadian bacon. Make a

big batch and freeze them individually for a quick and convenient breakfast option.

7. **Yogurt with Nuts and Seeds:** Plain Greek yogurt is low in sugar and high in protein, making it an excellent choice for stabilizing blood sugar levels. Top your yogurt with nuts, seeds, and a drizzle of honey or fruit for added flavor and texture.

8. **Vegetable and Bean Hash:** Sautee leftover vegetables and beans with spices such as cumin, chili powder, and paprika for a hearty and flavorful breakfast hash. Serve it with a side of scrambled eggs or whole grain toast for a complete meal.

Breakfast Meal Prep on a Budget

Meal prepping breakfast can save time and money during busy mornings while ensuring you have a nutritious meal ready to go. Here are some budget-friendly meal prep ideas for breakfast:

1. **Batch Cooking:** Cook large batches of breakfast staples such as oatmeal, quinoa, or breakfast burrito fillings on the weekend and portion them out for easy reheating throughout the week.

2. **Make-Ahead Smoothie Packs:** Prep individual smoothie packs by portioning out frozen fruit, leafy greens, and protein powder into resealable bags. In the morning, simply

dump the contents into a blender, add liquid, and blend until smooth.

3. **Overnight Oats:** Prepare individual servings of overnight oats in mason jars or resealable containers and store them in the refrigerator for up to several days. Customize each jar with different toppings and flavors for variety throughout the week.

4. **Egg Muffins:** Make a big batch of egg muffins filled with vegetables, cheese, and protein and store them in the refrigerator or freezer for a quick and easy breakfast option. Reheat them in the microwave or toaster oven for a convenient meal on busy mornings.

5. **Prep Ingredients in Advance:** Wash and chop fruits and vegetables in advance and store them in portioned containers in the refrigerator. This makes it easy to throw together a quick breakfast bowl or smoothie without any hassle.

6. **DIY Breakfast Sandwiches:** Assemble breakfast sandwiches using whole grain English muffins or bagels, eggs, cheese, and lean protein, and wrap them individually in foil or parchment paper. Store them in the refrigerator or freezer and reheat them in the microwave or toaster oven for a grab-and-go breakfast option.

7. **Homemade Granola:** Make your own granola at home using oats, nuts, seeds, and dried fruit. Store it in an airtight container and serve it with yogurt or milk for a quick and crunchy breakfast option.

8. **Portion Control:** Use portioned containers or resealable bags to portion out individual servings of breakfast items such as yogurt, granola, or smoothie ingredients for easy grab-and-go convenience.

By incorporating these simple and affordable breakfast ideas into your morning routine and utilizing meal prep strategies, you can enjoy nutritious and diabetes-friendly meals without breaking the bank. With a little planning and creativity, breakfast can become a delicious and stress-free part of your day.

CHAPTER FOUR

Economical Dinners for Every Night of the Week

Creating economical dinners that are both budget-friendly and delicious can be a challenge, especially when trying to manage diabetes. However, with the right recipes and strategies, it's possible to enjoy nutritious meals without breaking the bank. In this chapter, we'll explore one-pot meals for cost-effective cooking, budget-friendly sheet pan dinners, and quick and affordable stir-fries and skillet dishes that are perfect for any night of the week.

One-Pot Meals for Cost-Effective Cooking

One-pot meals are a lifesaver for busy weeknights—they require minimal prep and cleanup while delivering maximum flavor and nutrition. Here are some budget-friendly one-pot meal ideas:

1. **Vegetable Soup:** Whip up a big batch of vegetable soup using leftover vegetables, beans, and whole grains such as barley or quinoa. Add broth, herbs, and spices for flavor, and simmer until everything is tender and flavorful. Serve with a slice of whole grain bread for a complete meal.

2. **Chili:** Make a pot of hearty chili using beans, tomatoes, onions, and spices such as cumin, chili powder, and paprika. Add ground turkey or lean ground beef for extra protein, and

simmer until thick and flavorful. Serve with toppings such as cheese, sour cream, and avocado for a satisfying meal.

3. **Pasta Primavera:** Cook pasta with a variety of colorful vegetables such as bell peppers, zucchini, and cherry tomatoes for a quick and easy dinner. Toss with olive oil, garlic, and herbs such as basil and oregano for added flavor. Top with grated Parmesan cheese for a finishing touch.

4. **Rice and Beans:** Combine cooked rice with beans, vegetables, and spices for a simple and satisfying meal. Add protein such as chicken, tofu, or shrimp for extra flavor and nutrition. Serve with a side of salsa or guacamole for a Mexican-inspired twist.

5. **Quinoa Salad:** Cook quinoa and toss it with chopped vegetables, beans, and a flavorful dressing for a nutritious and filling dinner. Add protein such as grilled chicken or chickpeas for extra staying power. Serve chilled or at room temperature for a refreshing meal.

6. **Stuffed Peppers:** Fill bell peppers with a mixture of cooked rice, beans, vegetables, and cheese for a hearty and flavorful meal. Bake until the peppers are tender and the filling is heated through. Serve with a side of salsa or Greek yogurt for dipping.

7. **Curry:** Make a pot of curry using canned coconut milk, vegetables, and protein such as tofu or chickpeas for a flavorful and filling dinner. Add spices such as curry powder, turmeric, and ginger for depth of flavor. Serve with rice or naan bread for soaking up the sauce.

8. **Pulled Chicken or Pork:** Cook chicken or pork in a slow cooker with onions, garlic, and barbecue sauce for tender and flavorful meat that can be used in a variety of dishes. Serve on whole grain buns or wraps with coleslaw for a classic barbecue meal.

Budget-Friendly Sheet Pan Dinners

Sheet pan dinners are a convenient and economical way to cook a complete meal with minimal effort. Here are some budget-friendly sheet pan dinner ideas:

1. **Chicken and Vegetables:** Toss chicken breasts or thighs with vegetables such as broccoli, bell peppers, and onions in a simple marinade or seasoning blend. Roast on a sheet pan until the chicken is cooked through and the vegetables are tender and caramelized.

2. **Salmon and Asparagus:** Season salmon fillets with lemon juice, garlic, and herbs such as dill and parsley. Arrange on a sheet pan with asparagus spears and cherry tomatoes, and roast until the salmon is flaky and the vegetables are tender.

3. **Sausage and Potatoes:** Slice sausage links into coins and toss with cubed potatoes, onions, and bell peppers in a savory seasoning blend. Spread on a sheet pan and roast until the sausage is browned and the potatoes are crispy.

4. **Vegetable Fajitas:** Toss sliced bell peppers, onions, and mushrooms with fajita seasoning and olive oil on a sheet pan. Roast until the vegetables are tender and caramelized, then serve with warm tortillas, salsa, and guacamole for a delicious and filling meal.

5. **Pork and Brussels Sprouts:** Season pork tenderloin or chops with mustard, honey, and garlic, then arrange on a sheet pan with halved Brussels sprouts. Roast until the pork is cooked through and the Brussels sprouts are golden brown and crispy.

6. **Shrimp and Broccoli:** Toss shrimp with garlic, lemon juice, and red pepper flakes, then arrange on a sheet pan with broccoli florets. Roast until the shrimp are pink and opaque and the broccoli is tender and slightly charred.

7. **Tofu and Cauliflower:** Cube tofu and toss with a flavorful marinade or seasoning blend, then arrange on a sheet pan with cauliflower florets. Roast until the tofu is crispy and the cauliflower is golden brown and caramelized.

8. **Meatless Sheet Pan Dinner:** Combine a variety of vegetables such as sweet potatoes, carrots, and Brussels sprouts on a sheet pan with chickpeas or black beans. Season with herbs and spices, and roast until the vegetables are tender and the beans are crispy.

Quick and Affordable Stir-Fries and Skillet Dishes

Stir-fries and skillet dishes are quick, versatile, and budget-friendly, making them perfect for busy weeknights. Here are some ideas to get you started:

1. **Vegetable Stir-Fry:** Heat oil in a skillet and sauté chopped vegetables such as bell peppers, broccoli, and snap peas until tender-crisp. Add tofu or chicken for protein, and toss with a flavorful sauce such as teriyaki or ginger soy. Serve over rice or noodles for a complete meal.

2. **Beef and Broccoli:** Slice beef sirloin thinly and stir-fry with broccoli florets and sliced onions in a savory sauce made from soy sauce, garlic, and ginger. Serve over rice or noodles for a hearty and satisfying dinner.

3. **Chicken and Vegetable Skillet:** Brown chicken breasts or thighs in a skillet, then remove from the pan and set aside. Sauté sliced vegetables such as zucchini, bell peppers, and

onions until tender, then return the chicken to the pan and simmer in a flavorful sauce until cooked through.

4. **Shrimp Fried Rice:** Cook rice according to package instructions and let cool. Heat oil in a skillet and sauté cooked rice with shrimp, chopped vegetables, and scrambled eggs until heated through. Season with soy sauce and sesame oil for a quick and flavorful meal.

5. **Tofu and Vegetable Stir-Fry:** Cube tofu and stir-fry with a variety of vegetables such as bell peppers, snap peas, and carrots in a flavorful sauce made from soy sauce, garlic, and ginger. Serve over rice or noodles for a vegetarian-friendly meal.

6. **Pork and Cabbage Skillet:** Brown ground pork in a skillet with sliced cabbage, onions, and garlic until cooked through and caramelized. Season with soy sauce, ginger, and chili flakes for a flavorful and budget-friendly dinner.

7. **Vegetarian Chili Stir-Fry:** Sauté chopped vegetables such as bell peppers, onions, and mushrooms in a skillet with chili powder, cumin, and garlic until tender. Add canned beans and diced tomatoes, and simmer until heated through. Serve over rice or quinoa for a hearty and satisfying meal.

8. **Spicy Sausage and Pepper Skillet:** Sauté sliced sausage links with bell peppers, onions, and garlic in a skillet until

browned and caramelized. Season with paprika, cayenne pepper, and Italian herbs for a spicy and flavorful dinner.

By incorporating these economical dinner ideas into your meal rotation, you can enjoy delicious and nutritious meals every night of the week without breaking the bank. With a little planning and creativity, eating well on a budget is easier than you might think.

CHAPTER FIVE

Stretching Your Dollar with Sides and Accompaniments

Side dishes and accompaniments are an essential part of any meal, adding flavor, texture, and nutrition to the main course. However, they can also contribute to the overall cost of a meal. In this chapter, we'll explore how to stretch your dollar with inexpensive vegetable side dishes, budget-friendly grain and legume side dishes, and low-cost alternatives to traditional side dishes that won't break the bank.

Inexpensive Vegetable Side Dishes

Vegetables are a versatile and budget-friendly option for side dishes, offering a wide variety of flavors and textures. Here are some inexpensive vegetable side dishes to consider:

1. **Roasted Vegetables:** Toss chopped vegetables such as carrots, potatoes, and cauliflower with olive oil, salt, and pepper, then roast in the oven until tender and caramelized. Roasting brings out the natural sweetness of vegetables and enhances their flavor without the need for expensive seasonings or sauces.

2. **Steamed Vegetables:** Steam vegetables such as broccoli, green beans, and asparagus until tender-crisp, then toss with a squeeze of lemon juice and a sprinkle of salt and pepper

for a simple and healthy side dish. Steaming vegetables helps preserve their nutrients and vibrant color while keeping costs low.

3. **Stir-Fried Vegetables:** Stir-fry a mix of colorful vegetables such as bell peppers, snap peas, and mushrooms in a hot skillet with a splash of soy sauce and a sprinkle of sesame seeds for a quick and flavorful side dish. Stir-frying vegetables allows them to retain their crisp texture and vibrant color while adding depth of flavor.

4. **Vegetable Medley:** Combine a variety of vegetables such as zucchini, yellow squash, bell peppers, and cherry tomatoes in a baking dish with olive oil, garlic, and herbs such as thyme and rosemary. Roast in the oven until tender and golden brown for a delicious and visually appealing side dish.

5. **Coleslaw:** Make your own coleslaw using shredded cabbage, carrots, and onions tossed with a simple dressing made from mayonnaise, vinegar, and a touch of sugar. Coleslaw is a classic and budget-friendly side dish that pairs well with grilled meats and sandwiches.

6. **Sauteed Greens:** Sautee leafy greens such as spinach, kale, or Swiss chard in a hot skillet with garlic, olive oil, and a splash of lemon juice for a quick and nutritious side dish. Leafy greens are packed with vitamins and minerals and are an economical option for adding variety to your meals.

7. **Vegetable Soup:** Make a big pot of vegetable soup using leftover vegetables, beans, and broth for a hearty and comforting side dish. Use seasonal vegetables and herbs for maximum flavor and nutrition, and freeze any leftovers for future meals.

8. **Grilled Vegetables:** Grill vegetables such as eggplant, zucchini, and bell peppers on a hot grill until tender and charred for a smoky and flavorful side dish. Drizzle with balsamic glaze or pesto for extra flavor, or serve with a dollop of Greek yogurt for a creamy and tangy finish.

Budget-Friendly Grain and Legume Side Dishes

Grains and legumes are inexpensive pantry staples that can be used to create hearty and satisfying side dishes. Here are some budget-friendly options to consider:

1. **Rice Pilaf:** Cook rice with aromatics such as onions, garlic, and spices such as cumin and turmeric for a flavorful and fragrant side dish. Add vegetables such as peas, carrots, and bell peppers for extra color and nutrition.

2. **Quinoa Salad:** Cook quinoa and toss it with chopped vegetables, herbs, and a simple vinaigrette dressing for a light and refreshing side dish. Quinoa is a complete protein and pairs well with a variety of flavors and textures.

3. **Beans and Rice:** Combine cooked rice with canned beans, diced tomatoes, and spices such as chili powder and cumin for a quick and hearty side dish. Add vegetables such as corn, bell peppers, and onions for extra flavor and nutrition.

4. **Lentil Salad:** Cook lentils and toss them with diced vegetables, herbs, and a tangy dressing for a nutritious and filling side dish. Lentils are high in protein and fiber, making them a satisfying option for vegetarians and meat-eaters alike.

5. **Barley Risotto:** Cook barley with onions, garlic, and broth until tender and creamy for a delicious and budget-friendly side dish. Add vegetables such as mushrooms, peas, and carrots for extra flavor and nutrition.

6. **Black Bean Salad:** Combine canned black beans with corn, tomatoes, onions, and cilantro for a colorful and flavorful side dish. Dress with lime juice, olive oil, and spices such as cumin and chili powder for a Southwestern-inspired twist.

7. **Couscous Salad:** Cook couscous and toss it with diced vegetables, herbs, and a zesty dressing for a light and refreshing side dish. Couscous cooks quickly and pairs well with a variety of flavors and textures.

8. **Mashed Sweet Potatoes:** Cook sweet potatoes until tender, then mash them with butter, milk, and spices such as

cinnamon and nutmeg for a sweet and creamy side dish. Sweet potatoes are rich in vitamins and minerals and are an economical option for adding color and flavor to your meals.

Low-Cost Alternatives to Traditional Side Dishes

Traditional side dishes such as bread, potatoes, and pasta can be affordable, but there are also low-cost alternatives that offer variety and nutrition. Here are some options to consider:

1. **Whole Grain Bread:**Opt for whole grain bread instead of white bread for a healthier and more nutritious option. Whole grain bread is higher in fiber and vitamins and minerals than white bread and can be used to make sandwiches, toast, and croutons for salads.

2. **Sweet Potatoes:** Choose sweet potatoes over white potatoes for a nutrient-rich alternative that's lower in calories and higher in vitamins and minerals. Sweet potatoes can be baked, mashed, or roasted and are delicious served as a side dish or incorporated into recipes such as soups and stews.

3. **Zucchini Noodles:** Use spiralized zucchini noodles as a low-carb alternative to traditional pasta. Zucchini noodles are light and refreshing and can be tossed with sauces, vegetables, and proteins for a quick and healthy meal.

4. **Cauliflower Rice:** Swap cauliflower rice for traditional rice for a low-carb and low-calorie alternative that's rich in vitamins and minerals. Cauliflower rice can be used in stir-fries, pilafs, and grain bowls for a lighter and more nutritious option.

5. **Spaghetti Squash:** Cook spaghetti squash and use the strands as a substitute for traditional pasta. Spaghetti squash is low in calories and high in fiber and can be served with marinara sauce, pesto, or meatballs for a satisfying and nutritious meal.

6. **Lentil Pasta:** Choose lentil pasta or chickpea pasta over traditional wheat pasta for a gluten-free and protein-rich alternative. Lentil pasta is higher in fiber and lower in carbs than traditional pasta and can be used in a variety of pasta dishes for a nutritious and satisfying meal.

7. **Brown Rice:**Opt for brown rice instead of white rice for a whole grain alternative that's higher in fiber and nutrients. Brown rice can be served as a side dish or used in recipes such as stir-fries, pilafs, and salads for added nutrition and flavor.

8. **Quinoa:** Cook quinoa and use it as a versatile and nutritious alternative to grains such as rice and pasta. Quinoa is high in protein and fiber and can be used in salads, soups, casseroles, and pilafs for added texture and nutrition.

By incorporating these inexpensive side dishes and accompaniments into your meals, you can stretch your dollar while still enjoying delicious and nutritious meals. With a little creativity and planning, eating well on a budget is easy and satisfying.

CHAPTER SIX

Thrifty Desserts and Sweet Treats

Desserts and sweet treats are often considered indulgences, but they don't have to break the bank. With a little creativity and resourcefulness, it's possible to enjoy delicious desserts without spending a fortune. In this chapter, we'll explore sugar-free dessert recipes for affordable indulgence, fruit-based desserts that are budget-friendly and delicious, and tips for baking on a budget without sacrificing flavor.

Sugar-Free Dessert Recipes for Affordable Indulgence

Sugar-free desserts are not only healthier but can also be more budget-friendly, as they often rely on natural sweeteners and fewer ingredients. Here are some sugar-free dessert recipes to satisfy your sweet tooth without breaking the bank:

1. **Sugar-Free Banana Bread:** Make a batch of sugar-free banana bread using ripe bananas, whole wheat flour, eggs, and a touch of honey or maple syrup for sweetness. Add nuts or seeds for extra texture and flavor, and enjoy a guilt-free treat any time of day.

2. **Stevia-Sweetened Brownies:** Whip up a batch of stevia-sweetened brownies using cocoa powder, almond flour, eggs, and a natural sweetener such as stevia or erythritol.

These brownies are rich, fudgy, and satisfying without the added sugar.

3. **No-Bake Energy Bites:** Mix together oats, nut butter, honey or maple syrup, and add-ins such as nuts, seeds, and dried fruit to create no-bake energy bites that are perfect for a quick and healthy dessert or snack. Customize the recipe to suit your taste preferences and enjoy a sweet treat on the go.

4. **Greek Yogurt Parfait:** Layer Greek yogurt with fresh berries, nuts, and a drizzle of honey or agave nectar for a creamy and indulgent dessert that's high in protein and low in sugar. Experiment with different fruit and nut combinations for variety.

5. **Chia Seed Pudding:** Make chia seed pudding by combining chia seeds with milk or non-dairy milk, vanilla extract, and a natural sweetener such as honey or maple syrup. Let it sit in the refrigerator overnight to thicken, then top with fresh fruit or nuts for a nutritious and satisfying dessert.

6. **Sugar-Free Apple Crisp:** Bake a sugar-free apple crisp using sliced apples, oats, cinnamon, and a touch of honey or agave nectar for sweetness. Top with a crunchy oat and nut topping and bake until golden brown and bubbly for a comforting and delicious dessert.

7. **Coconut Flour Cookies:** Bake coconut flour cookies using coconut flour, eggs, coconut oil, and a natural sweetener such as stevia or erythritol. Add chocolate chips or nuts for extra flavor and texture, and enjoy a guilt-free treat that's perfect for any occasion.

8. **Frozen Yogurt Bark:** Spread Greek yogurt onto a baking sheet and top with fruit, nuts, and a drizzle of honey or maple syrup. Freeze until solid, then break into pieces for a refreshing and nutritious dessert that's perfect for hot summer days.

Fruit-Based Desserts: Budget-Friendly and Delicious

Fruits are naturally sweet and packed with vitamins, minerals, and fiber, making them an excellent choice for budget-friendly desserts. Here are some fruit-based dessert ideas to satisfy your sweet cravings without breaking the bank:

1. **Fruit Salad:** Combine a variety of fresh fruits such as berries, melons, grapes, and citrus fruits in a bowl for a colorful and refreshing dessert. Add a squeeze of lemon or lime juice and a sprinkle of mint for extra flavor, and enjoy a healthy and satisfying treat.

2. **Baked Apples:** Core apples and fill them with a mixture of oats, nuts, cinnamon, and a touch of honey or maple syrup.

Bake until tender and golden brown for a warm and comforting dessert that's perfect for fall.

3. **Grilled Pineapple:** Grill pineapple slices until caramelized and slightly charred for a sweet and smoky dessert that's perfect for summer cookouts. Serve with a dollop of Greek yogurt or a sprinkle of cinnamon for extra flavor.

4. **Frozen Fruit Pops:** Blend together your favorite fruits such as berries, mangoes, or peaches with yogurt or coconut milk, and pour into popsicle molds. Freeze until solid, then enjoy a refreshing and healthy dessert on a hot day.

5. **Fruit Crumble:** Combine sliced fruit such as berries, peaches, or apples with a crumbly topping made from oats, flour, butter, and a touch of honey or maple syrup. Bake until bubbly and golden brown for a comforting and delicious dessert that's perfect for sharing.

6. **Banana Nice Cream:** Freeze ripe bananas, then blend them in a food processor until smooth and creamy for a dairy-free and naturally sweet dessert. Add cocoa powder, peanut butter, or fruit for extra flavor, and enjoy a guilt-free treat any time of day.

7. **Fruit Salsa with Cinnamon Chips:** Dice a variety of fruits such as strawberries, kiwi, and mangoes and toss with a squeeze of lime juice and a sprinkle of cinnamon for a flavorful and

colorful dessert salsa. Serve with homemade cinnamon chips made from flour tortillas for dipping.

8. **Baked Pears:** Halve pears and remove the cores, then fill them with a mixture of oats, nuts, cinnamon, and a touch of honey or maple syrup. Bake until tender and golden brown for a warm and comforting dessert that's perfect for chilly nights.

Tips for Baking on a Budget without Sacrificing Flavor

Baking can be a cost-effective way to satisfy your sweet tooth, but it's essential to be mindful of your budget. Here are some tips for baking on a budget without sacrificing flavor:

1. **Use Basic Ingredients:** Stick to basic ingredients such as flour, sugar, eggs, and butter for simple and budget-friendly baked goods. Avoid specialty ingredients that can be expensive and opt for pantry staples instead.

2. **Buy in Bulk:** Purchase baking staples such as flour, sugar, and oats in bulk to save money in the long run. Look for discounts on large bags or containers at warehouse clubs or bulk food stores, and store extras in airtight containers for future use.

3. **Shop Sales and Discounts:** Keep an eye out for sales and discounts on baking ingredients at your local grocery store or

online. Stock up on items when they're on sale and freeze them for later use to take advantage of lower prices.

4. **Use Seasonal Produce:** Incorporate seasonal fruits and vegetables into your baked goods to take advantage of lower prices and better flavor. Visit farmers' markets or pick-your-own farms to find fresh produce at competitive prices and use them in recipes such as pies, crisps, and muffins.

5. **Make Your Own Mixes:** Skip pre-packaged baking mixes and make your own at home using basic ingredients such as flour, baking powder, and salt. Mix up a big batch and store it in an airtight container for quick and easy baking whenever the mood strikes.

6. **Substitute Ingredients:** Get creative with ingredient substitutions to save money and reduce waste. For example, use applesauce or mashed bananas instead of oil or butter in recipes, or swap out expensive nuts and seeds for cheaper alternatives such as sunflower or pumpkin seeds.

7. **Use Leftover Ingredients:** Make the most of leftover ingredients by incorporating them into your baking. For example, use leftover fruit to make muffins or bread, or add nuts and chocolate chips to cookies and bars for extra flavor and texture.

8. **Portion Control:** Be mindful of portion sizes when baking to avoid waste and save money. Cut larger recipes in half or freeze individual portions for later use to prevent leftovers from going to waste.

By incorporating these thrifty dessert ideas and budget-friendly baking tips into your routine, you can satisfy your sweet tooth without breaking the bank. With a little creativity and resourcefulness, delicious desserts are within reach, no matter your budget.

CHAPTER SEVEN

Budget-Friendly Tips for Dining Out with Diabetes

Dining out with diabetes can present unique challenges, but with careful planning and smart choices, it's possible to enjoy delicious meals at restaurants without compromising your health or budget. In this chapter, we'll explore budget-friendly tips for dining out with diabetes, including strategies for eating out healthily without breaking the bank, making smart menu choices on a budget at restaurants, and navigating social situations and special occasions without overspending.

Strategies for Eating Out Healthily Without Breaking the Bank

Eating out healthily doesn't have to be expensive. With these strategies, you can enjoy meals at restaurants while sticking to your budget and managing your diabetes:

1. **Plan Ahead:** Before dining out, research restaurants in your area that offer healthy options at affordable prices. Look for menus online and read reviews to find restaurants that cater to dietary needs and preferences.

2. **Set a Budget:** Decide on a budget for dining out and stick to it. Consider factors such as the cost of the meal, drinks, tax,

and tip, and choose restaurants that fit within your budget while still offering nutritious options.

3. **Choose Wisely:**Opt for restaurants that offer a variety of healthy choices, such as salads, grilled meats, and steamed vegetables. Avoid fast food and chain restaurants that may have limited options or oversized portions.

4. **Share Meals:** Consider sharing a meal with a friend or family member to save money and reduce food waste. Many restaurants offer large portions that can be split between two people, allowing you to enjoy a satisfying meal without overeating or overspending.

5. **Skip the Extras:** Avoid ordering appetizers, desserts, and alcoholic beverages, which can add extra calories and cost to your meal. Stick to water or unsweetened beverages to save money and stay hydrated.

6. **Ask for Substitutions:** Don't be afraid to ask for substitutions or modifications to accommodate your dietary needs. Request steamed vegetables instead of fries, whole grain bread instead of white, or dressing on the side to control portions and calories.

7. **Be Mindful of Portions:** Pay attention to portion sizes and listen to your body's hunger and fullness cues. Eat slowly,

savoring each bite, and stop when you feel satisfied, rather than stuffed.

8. **Take leftovers home:** If you're unable to finish your meal, ask for a takeout container and bring the leftovers home. Leftovers can be enjoyed for lunch or dinner the next day, saving you money and preventing food waste.

Making Smart Menu Choices on a Budget at Restaurants

When dining out on a budget, it's important to make smart menu choices that are both affordable and diabetes-friendly. Here are some tips for navigating restaurant menus while sticking to your budget:

1. **Focus on Protein:** Look for menu items that are high in protein and low in carbohydrates, such as grilled chicken, fish, or lean beef. Protein-rich foods can help keep you feeling full and satisfied without causing spikes in blood sugar levels.

2. **Load Up on Vegetables:** Choose dishes that are loaded with vegetables, such as salads, stir-fries, or vegetable-based soups. Vegetables are low in calories and carbohydrates, making them an excellent choice for managing diabetes and staying within your budget.

3. **Watch for Hidden Sugars:** Be wary of dishes that may contain hidden sugars, such as sauces, dressings, and marinades. Ask your server for information about ingredients and preparation methods to ensure that your meal aligns with your dietary needs.

4. **Avoid Fried Foods:** Steer clear of fried foods, which are often high in unhealthy fats and calories. Instead, choose grilled, baked, or steamed options that are lower in fat and more diabetes-friendly.

5. **Read the Fine Print:** Pay attention to menu descriptions and nutritional information, if available, to make informed choices about your meal. Look for keywords such as "grilled," "steamed," or "baked," which indicate healthier cooking methods.

6. **Choose Whole Grains:**Opt for whole grain options such as brown rice, quinoa, or whole wheat pasta, which are higher in fiber and nutrients than refined grains. Whole grains can help stabilize blood sugar levels and promote overall health.

7. **BYO Dressing:** Consider bringing your own salad dressing or condiments to restaurants to avoid added sugars and unhealthy fats. Pack a small container of olive oil and vinegar, lemon juice, or low-sugar dressing to dress your salad or vegetables.

8. **Think Outside the Box:** Don't be afraid to think outside the box and customize your meal to suit your dietary needs and preferences. Ask for substitutions or modifications to make dishes more diabetes-friendly and budget-friendly.

Navigating Social Situations and Special Occasions on a Budget

Social situations and special occasions can present challenges when dining out with diabetes, but with these tips, you can navigate them with confidence and ease:

1. **Communicate Your Needs:** Be upfront with friends, family members, and restaurant staff about your dietary needs and preferences. Let them know that you're managing diabetes and may need to make special requests or modifications to your meal.

2. **Offer to Host:** Consider hosting social gatherings or special occasions at home to save money and have more control over the menu. Prepare diabetes-friendly dishes that everyone can enjoy, and encourage guests to bring a dish to share to lighten the load and reduce costs.

3. **Plan Ahead:** If you're attending a social event or special occasion at a restaurant, review the menu ahead of time and decide on a few options that fit within your budget and

dietary needs. This will help you make a quick and confident decision when it's time to order.

4. **Eat Before You Go:** If you're worried about finding diabetes-friendly options at a social event or special occasion, consider eating a small, balanced meal or snack before you go. This will help prevent overeating or making unhealthy choices when you arrive.

5. **Focus on Socializing:** Remember that social gatherings and special occasions are about more than just food. Focus on enjoying the company of friends and loved ones rather than fixating on what you can or can't eat.

6. **Be Prepared:** Carry snacks with you when you're out and about to prevent low blood sugar levels and avoid the temptation of unhealthy options. Pack portable snacks such as nuts, seeds, fruit, or whole grain crackers to keep you fueled and satisfied.

7. **Stay Flexible:** Be flexible and open-minded when dining out with others, and don't be afraid to adapt or modify your meal to fit your dietary needs. Look for creative solutions and compromises that allow everyone to enjoy the experience without compromising their health or budget.

8. **Practice Self-Care:** Finally, remember to prioritize self-care and listen to your body's needs. If you're feeling stressed or

overwhelmed, take a step back and focus on activities that bring you joy and relaxation, such as exercise, meditation, or spending time outdoors.

By following these budget-friendly tips for dining out with diabetes, you can enjoy delicious meals at restaurants without compromising your health or breaking the bank. With a little planning and creativity, dining out can be a fun and enjoyable experience that supports your overall well-being.

CHAPTER EIGHT

Budget-Friendly Meal Prep for Diabetes Management

Meal prep is a powerful tool for managing diabetes while sticking to a budget. By planning and preparing your meals ahead of time, you can save money, control portion sizes, and make healthier choices. In this chapter, we'll explore budget-friendly meal prep for diabetes management, including an introduction to meal prep on a budget, strategies for batch cooking to maximize efficiency and minimize waste, and budget-friendly meal prep recipes for busy weekdays.

Introduction to Meal Prep for Diabetes on a Budget

Meal prep involves planning and preparing meals in advance to make eating healthier and more convenient. When managing diabetes on a budget, meal prep becomes even more essential as it allows you to control portion sizes, choose nutritious ingredients, and save money by avoiding impulse purchases or dining out. Here are some key principles for meal prepping on a budget:

1. **Plan Ahead:** Start by creating a weekly meal plan that includes breakfast, lunch, dinner, and snacks. Consider your dietary needs, preferences, and budget when selecting

recipes and ingredients. Planning ahead helps you stay organized and prevents last-minute trips to the grocery store.

2. **Shop Smart:** Make a list of ingredients based on your meal plan and stick to it when shopping. Look for sales, discounts, and coupons to save money on staple items such as grains, proteins, and produce. Consider buying in bulk or choosing store-brand products to stretch your dollars further.

3. **Use Leftovers:** Embrace leftovers as a budget-friendly way to make the most of your meals. Cook larger batches of food and portion them out into individual containers for easy grab-and-go meals throughout the week. Leftovers can also be repurposed into new dishes to reduce food waste.

4. **Focus on Staples:** Stock your pantry with staple ingredients such as whole grains, beans, canned tomatoes, and spices that can be used to create a variety of meals. These budget-friendly staples form the foundation of many recipes and can be customized based on what's on sale or in season.

5. **Choose Affordable Proteins:** Protein can be one of the most expensive components of a meal, but there are plenty of budget-friendly options to choose from. Consider incorporating plant-based proteins such as beans, lentils, tofu, or eggs into your meals to save money without sacrificing nutrition.

6. **Minimize Waste:** Be mindful of food waste by using up ingredients before they spoil and repurposing leftovers into new dishes. Get creative with meal planning to use ingredients in multiple meals throughout the week, and freeze extra portions for later use.

7. **Invest in Quality Containers:** Invest in a set of high-quality, reusable containers for storing and transporting your prepped meals. Choose containers that are durable, leak-proof, and microwave-safe for easy reheating and cleaning. Investing in quality containers upfront can save you money in the long run by reducing the need for disposable alternatives.

8. **Stay Flexible:** Stay flexible and open-minded with your meal prep approach, and don't be afraid to adjust your plans based on your schedule, budget, or dietary needs. Experiment with different recipes, ingredients, and cooking methods to find what works best for you.

Batch Cooking: Maximizing Efficiency and Minimizing Waste

Batch cooking is a meal prep strategy that involves cooking large quantities of food at once and portioning it out into individual servings for later use. Batch cooking is a cost-effective way to save time, money, and energy while ensuring that you always have healthy meals on hand. Here are some tips for maximizing efficiency and minimizing waste with batch cooking:

1. **Choose Versatile Recipes:** Select recipes that can be easily scaled up to make large batches without sacrificing flavor or quality. Choose versatile ingredients that can be used in multiple dishes throughout the week to minimize waste and maximize efficiency.

2. **Plan Your Menu:** Create a weekly menu that includes batch-friendly recipes for breakfast, lunch, dinner, and snacks. Consider recipes that use similar ingredients to streamline your shopping list and minimize waste. Focus on one-pot meals, casseroles, soups, and stews that can be easily batch cooked and portioned out for later use.

3. **Schedule a Cooking Day:** Set aside a dedicated day each week for batch cooking and meal prep. Use this time to cook large batches of food, portion out individual servings, and store them in the refrigerator or freezer for later use. Involve family members or friends to make the process more enjoyable and efficient.

4. **Invest in Time-Saving Appliances:** Invest in time-saving appliances such as a slow cooker, Instant Pot, or air fryer to streamline the batch cooking process. These appliances allow you to cook large quantities of food with minimal hands-on time, making meal prep easier and more efficient.

5. **Portion Out Meals:** Once your batch-cooked meals are ready, portion them out into individual containers for easy

grab-and-go meals throughout the week. Label containers with the date and contents to keep track of what's in your fridge or freezer and prevent food waste.

6. **Get Creative with Leftovers:** Use leftover ingredients from batch cooking to create new dishes and reduce food waste. Repurpose cooked grains, proteins, and vegetables into salads, stir-fries, sandwiches, or grain bowls for quick and easy meals. Get creative with spices, sauces, and seasonings to change up the flavors and keep things interesting.

7. **Freeze Extra Portions:** If you have leftover batch-cooked meals that you won't be able to eat within a few days, freeze them for later use. Use freezer-safe containers or resealable bags to store individual portions of soups, stews, casseroles, or sauces for up to several months. Thaw frozen meals in the refrigerator overnight or reheat them directly from frozen for a convenient and budget-friendly option.

8. **Plan for Variety:** While batch cooking can save time and money, it's essential to plan for variety to prevent boredom and ensure balanced nutrition. Mix and match batch-cooked meals with fresh salads, sandwiches, or wraps for a diverse and satisfying meal plan that meets your dietary needs and preferences.

CHAPTER NINE

Budget-Friendly Meal Prep Recipes for Busy Weekdays

Preparing budget-friendly meal prep recipes ahead of time can save you time and money during busy weekdays. Here are some nutritious and delicious recipes that are perfect for meal prep:

1. **Vegetable Stir-Fry:** Whip up a large batch of vegetable stir-fry using a mix of colorful vegetables such as bell peppers, broccoli, carrots, and snap peas. Stir-fry the vegetables in a hot skillet with garlic, ginger, and your favorite stir-fry sauce until tender-crisp. Serve over cooked brown rice or quinoa for a satisfying and nutritious meal.

2. **Turkey and Black Bean Chili:** Make a big pot of turkey and black bean chili using lean ground turkey, black beans, tomatoes, onions, and spices such as chili powder, cumin, and paprika. Let the chili simmer on the stove or in a slow cooker until thick and flavorful, then portion it out into individual containers for easy lunches or dinners throughout the week. Top with Greek yogurt, shredded cheese, and chopped green onions for extra flavor and texture.

3. **Quinoa Salad with Roasted Vegetables:** Cook a batch of quinoa and toss it with roasted vegetables such as sweet potatoes, Brussels sprouts, and cauliflower. Add canned

chickpeas or black beans for protein, and drizzle with a simple vinaigrette made from olive oil, lemon juice, and herbs such as parsley and thyme. Serve the quinoa salad cold or at room temperature for a refreshing and nutritious meal that's perfect for lunch or dinner.

4. **Chicken and Vegetable Sheet Pan Dinner:** Sheet pan dinners are a convenient and budget-friendly option for meal prep. Arrange chicken breasts or thighs on a baking sheet with a mix of chopped vegetables such as potatoes, carrots, and green beans. Drizzle with olive oil and season with herbs and spices such as rosemary, thyme, and garlic powder. Roast in the oven until the chicken is cooked through and the vegetables are tender and caramelized. Divide into individual servings and store in the refrigerator for easy reheating during the week.

5. **Egg Muffin Cups:** Whip up a batch of egg muffin cups using eggs, vegetables, and cheese. Beat eggs in a large bowl and stir in diced vegetables such as bell peppers, spinach, onions, and tomatoes. Pour the egg mixture into greased muffin tins and sprinkle with shredded cheese. Bake in the oven until the eggs are set and the muffins are golden brown. Let cool, then portion out into individual containers for a quick and portable breakfast option that's perfect for busy mornings.

6. **Salmon and Quinoa Bowls:** Cook a batch of quinoa and grill or bake salmon fillets until cooked through. Divide the quinoa and salmon into individual containers and add steamed vegetables such as broccoli, green beans, and carrots. Drizzle with a tangy yogurt sauce made from Greek yogurt, lemon juice, garlic, and dill for a flavorful and nutritious meal that's packed with protein and fiber.

7. **Vegetable Soup:** Make a big pot of vegetable soup using seasonal vegetables such as carrots, celery, onions, and potatoes. Add canned tomatoes, vegetable broth, and herbs such as thyme, oregano, and bay leaves for flavor. Let the soup simmer on the stove until the vegetables are tender and the flavors have melded together. Divide into individual containers and store in the refrigerator or freezer for a comforting and nourishing meal that's perfect for chilly days.

8. **Black Bean and Corn Salad:** Combine canned black beans, corn, diced tomatoes, onions, and bell peppers in a large bowl. Toss with lime juice, olive oil, and spices such as cumin, chili powder, and cilantro for a zesty and flavorful salad that's perfect for meal prep. Serve the black bean and corn salad cold or at room temperature as a side dish or light lunch option.

By incorporating these budget-friendly meal prep strategies and recipes into your routine, you can save time, money, and energy while managing your diabetes effectively. With a little planning and preparation, you can enjoy delicious and nutritious meals every day without breaking the bank.

CHAPTER TEN

Building Sustainable Budget-Friendly Habits

Creating sustainable budget-friendly habits is essential for long-term success in managing diabetes while also maintaining financial stability. In this chapter, we'll delve into setting realistic budget goals for diabetes management, overcoming challenges in eating healthy on a budget, and celebrating successes while sustaining budget-friendly practices.

Setting Realistic Budget Goals for Diabetes Management

When managing diabetes, setting realistic budget goals is crucial for ensuring that your financial resources align with your health needs. Here are some steps to help you set achievable budget goals:

1. **Assess Your Current Expenses:** Start by examining your current spending habits to identify areas where you can make adjustments. Look for opportunities to cut back on non-essential expenses such as dining out, entertainment, or luxury items, and reallocate those funds towards healthier food choices and diabetes management expenses.

2. **Calculate Your Monthly Budget:** Determine how much you can realistically afford to allocate towards groceries, meal prep, medications, and other diabetes-related expenses each

month. Consider factors such as your income, savings, debt, and other financial obligations when setting your budget goals.

3. **Prioritize Your Health:** Recognize that investing in your health is a priority, and allocate a portion of your budget towards nutritious food, regular exercise, and medical expenses related to diabetes management. Remember that prevention and early intervention can help reduce the long-term costs associated with diabetes complications.

4. **Set Specific and Measurable Goals:** Set specific and measurable goals for your budget, such as reducing your monthly grocery bill by a certain percentage or increasing your savings for diabetes medications and supplies. Break down your goals into smaller, achievable milestones to track your progress over time.

5. **Adjust as Needed:** Be flexible and willing to adjust your budget goals as needed based on changes in your financial situation or health needs. Reevaluate your budget regularly and make adjustments as necessary to ensure that it remains realistic and sustainable in the long term.

6. **Seek Support:** Don't be afraid to seek support from family members, friends, or healthcare professionals when setting and achieving your budget goals. Consider joining support

groups or online communities for individuals with diabetes to share tips, resources, and encouragement along the way.

7. **Celebrate Progress:** Celebrate your progress and achievements as you work towards your budget goals. Recognize and reward yourself for reaching milestones, such as sticking to your budget for a certain period of time or successfully implementing cost-saving strategies in your daily life.

8. **Stay Positive and Persistent:** Stay positive and persistent in your efforts to manage your diabetes and stick to your budget goals. Remember that building sustainable habits takes time and effort, but the rewards of improved health and financial well-being are well worth it in the end.

Overcoming Challenges in Eating Healthy on a Budget

Eating healthy on a budget can present unique challenges, but with the right strategies and mindset, it's entirely achievable. Here are some common challenges and tips for overcoming them:

1. **Limited Access to Affordable Foods:** If you live in an area with limited access to affordable fresh produce or healthy food options, explore alternative shopping options such as farmers' markets, community gardens, or food cooperatives. Consider joining a community-supported agriculture (CSA)

program to receive fresh, locally grown produce at a discounted price.

2. **Time Constraints:** Balancing work, family, and other responsibilities can make it challenging to find time for meal planning, shopping, and cooking. To overcome this challenge, prioritize meal prep and planning by scheduling dedicated time each week to plan your meals, create a shopping list, and prepare ingredients in advance. Consider batch cooking and freezing meals to save time during busy weekdays.

3. **Food Waste:** Food waste can be a significant drain on your budget and contribute to environmental waste. To minimize food waste, plan your meals carefully to use up ingredients before they spoil, store leftovers in airtight containers for future use, and repurpose scraps and leftovers into new dishes. Composting can also help reduce food waste while enriching soil for gardening.

4. **Temptation to Eat Out:** The convenience and allure of dining out can make it tempting to stray from your budget and healthy eating goals. Combat this temptation by planning ahead and bringing homemade meals or snacks with you when you're on the go. Choose restaurants that offer affordable and nutritious options, and opt for water or unsweetened beverages to save money on drinks.

5. **Lack of Cooking Skills:** If you're not confident in your cooking skills, start by mastering a few simple recipes and gradually expand your repertoire over time. Take advantage of free resources such as cooking classes, online tutorials, and cookbooks to learn new techniques and recipes. Cooking with friends or family members can also make the experience more enjoyable and educational.

6. **Unrealistic Expectations:** Setting unrealistic expectations for yourself can lead to frustration and burnout. Be gentle with yourself and recognize that building healthy eating habits takes time and practice. Focus on making small, sustainable changes to your diet and lifestyle, and celebrate progress no matter how small.

7. **Social Pressures:** Social situations such as dining out with friends or attending parties can make it challenging to stick to your budget and healthy eating goals. Communicate your dietary needs and preferences to friends and family members, and seek out supportive social environments that encourage and facilitate healthy choices. Offer to host gatherings at your home and prepare budget-friendly, diabetes-friendly meals for your guests to enjoy.

8. **Lack of Motivation:** Lack of motivation or willpower can derail your efforts to eat healthy on a budget. Find sources of inspiration and motivation that resonate with you,

whether it's setting specific health goals, tracking your progress, or seeking support from others. Focus on the positive benefits of healthy eating, such as improved energy, mood, and overall well-being, to stay motivated and committed to your goals.

Celebrating Successes and Sustaining Budget-Friendly Practices

Celebrating successes and sustaining budget-friendly practices are essential for maintaining motivation and momentum in managing your diabetes and finances. Here are some tips for celebrating successes and sustaining healthy habits:

1. **Acknowledge Achievements:** Take time to acknowledge and celebrate your achievements, no matter how small. Whether it's sticking to your budget for a week, reaching a milestone in your health goals, or mastering a new cooking technique, recognize your efforts and give yourself credit for your accomplishments.

2. **Reward Yourself:** Reward yourself for reaching milestones and achieving your goals. Treat yourself to a small indulgence or a special activity that brings you joy and relaxation. Choose rewards that align with your health and financial goals, such as a healthy meal at your favorite restaurant or a day of outdoor activities.

3. **Reflect on Progress:** Reflect on your progress regularly and celebrate the positive changes you've made in your life. Keep a journal or log to track your achievements, milestones, and challenges, and use it as a source of inspiration and motivation during difficult times. Share your successes with friends, family members, or support groups to receive encouragement and validation.

4. **Stay Connected:** Stay connected with others who share similar goals and challenges related to diabetes management and budget-friendly living. Join support groups or online communities to share tips, resources, and experiences, and offer support and encouragement to others on their journey. Building a supportive network of like-minded individuals can help you stay motivated and accountable in reaching your goals.

5. **Set New Goals:** Once you've achieved your initial goals, set new ones to continue challenging yourself and pushing your limits. Set specific, measurable, and achievable goals that align with your values and priorities, and break them down into smaller milestones to track your progress over time. Keep pushing yourself to grow and improve, and celebrate each step along the way.

6. **Stay Flexible:** Be flexible and adaptable in your approach to managing your diabetes and finances. Life is unpredictable,

and unexpected challenges or setbacks may arise along the way. Stay open-minded and willing to adjust your goals and strategies as needed to overcome obstacles and stay on track towards your desired outcomes.

7. **Practice Gratitude:** Cultivate a sense of gratitude for the progress you've made and the resources you have available to you. Focus on the positive aspects of your life and the things that bring you joy, fulfillment, and meaning. Practice gratitude daily by expressing appreciation for the people, experiences, and opportunities that enrich your life and contribute to your well-being.

8. **Celebrate Milestones:** Celebrate important milestones and anniversaries in your journey towards better health and financial stability. Whether it's marking one year of sticking to your budget, reaching a significant weight loss goal, or achieving better blood sugar control, take time to celebrate your accomplishments and acknowledge the hard work and dedication it took to get there.

By setting realistic budget goals, overcoming challenges in eating healthy on a budget, and celebrating successes while sustaining budget-friendly practices, you can build sustainable habits that support your overall well-being and happiness. Remember that managing diabetes and maintaining financial stability are ongoing processes that require commitment, patience, and perseverance.

With determination and resilience, you can achieve your goals and live a fulfilling life with diabetes while staying within your budget.

CHAPTER 11

BONUS: SOME ESSENTIAL DIETS TO KNOW

TLC Diet (Therapeutic Lifestyle Changes):

Definition:

The TLC diet is a heart-healthy eating plan designed to reduce cholesterol levels and lower the risk of heart disease. It emphasizes reducing intake of saturated fat and dietary cholesterol while focusing on consuming a variety of nutrient-rich foods, including fruits, vegetables, whole grains, lean proteins, and healthy fats. The diet also encourages regular physical activity and other lifestyle modifications to promote heart health.

Ingredients:

- Fruits: Berries, apples, oranges, bananas, grapes, etc.

- Vegetables: Leafy greens, broccoli, carrots, bell peppers, tomatoes, etc.

- Whole Grains: Oats, barley, quinoa, brown rice, whole wheat bread, whole grain pasta.

- Lean Proteins: Skinless poultry, fish, seafood, tofu, beans, lentils.

- Healthy Fats: Avocado, nuts, seeds, olive oil, fatty fish like salmon.

- Low-Fat or Fat-Free Dairy: Skim milk, low-fat yogurt, reduced-fat cheese.

- Herbs and Spices: Basil, oregano, garlic, turmeric, cinnamon, etc.

Instructions/How to Prepare:

1. Limit intake of saturated fats, trans fats, and dietary cholesterol by choosing lean proteins, low-fat dairy products, and healthy fats.

2. Focus on consuming a variety of colorful fruits and vegetables for essential vitamins, minerals, and antioxidants.

3. Choose whole grains over refined grains for added fiber and nutrients.

4. Incorporate lean proteins such as poultry, fish, tofu, beans, and lentils into meals and snacks.

5. Use healthy fats like avocado, nuts, seeds, and olive oil for cooking and dressing.

6. Limit consumption of processed foods, sugary snacks, and high-fat meats.

7. Be mindful of portion sizes to avoid overeating, especially with calorie-dense foods.

8. Read food labels to identify hidden sources of saturated and trans fats, sodium, and added sugars.

9. Stay hydrated by drinking plenty of water throughout the day.

10.   Engage in regular physical activity, aiming for at least 30 minutes of moderate exercise most days of the week to complement dietary changes and promote overall heart health.

FODMAP Diet (Fermentable Oligosaccharides, Disaccharides, Monosaccharides, and Polyols):

Definition:

The FODMAP diet is a therapeutic approach to managing symptoms of irritable bowel syndrome (IBS) and other gastrointestinal disorders. It involves temporarily reducing or eliminating certain types of carbohydrates that are poorly absorbed in the small intestine and can ferment in the colon, leading to gas, bloating, abdominal pain, and other digestive symptoms. The diet consists of three phases: elimination, reintroduction, and personalization.

Ingredients:

- Low-FODMAP Fruits: Berries, citrus fruits, bananas, grapes, kiwi, etc.

- Low-FODMAP Vegetables: Leafy greens, carrots, bell peppers, zucchini, potatoes, etc.

- Low-FODMAP Grains: Quinoa, rice (white and brown), oats (gluten-free), etc.

- Low-FODMAP Proteins: Chicken, turkey, fish, eggs, tofu, tempeh, firm tofu, etc.

- Low-FODMAP Dairy: Lactose-free milk, lactose-free yogurt, hard cheeses (e.g., cheddar), etc.

- Low-FODMAP Fats and Oils: Olive oil, coconut oil, butter (in moderation), etc.

- Herbs and Spices: Basil, oregano, ginger, turmeric, cinnamon, etc.

Instructions/How to Prepare:

1. Start with the elimination phase, during which high-FODMAP foods are eliminated from the diet for 2-6 weeks to reduce symptoms.

2. Base meals around low-FODMAP foods such as fruits, vegetables, grains, proteins, and fats that are well-tolerated.

3. Gradually reintroduce high-FODMAP foods one at a time in small portions to identify trigger foods and tolerance levels.

4. Keep a food and symptom diary to track reactions to specific foods and help identify patterns.

5. Personalize the diet by incorporating a variety of low-FODMAP foods that are well-tolerated and avoiding or limiting high-FODMAP foods that trigger symptoms.

6. Be mindful of portion sizes and avoid overeating, as consuming large quantities of even low-FODMAP foods can exacerbate symptoms.

7. Consider working with a registered dietitian experienced in the FODMAP diet to ensure proper implementation and guidance throughout the process.

8. Stay hydrated by drinking plenty of water throughout the day to support digestive health.

9. Experiment with cooking methods and recipes to add flavor and variety to meals while adhering to the low-FODMAP guidelines.

10.   Monitor symptoms regularly and adjust your diet as needed to manage symptoms effectively and improve overall quality of life.

Pescatarian Diet:

Definition:

The piscatorial diet is a plant-based eating pattern that includes fish and seafood but excludes other animal meats such as poultry, beef, and pork. It's a flexible approach to eating that emphasizes plant foods such as fruits, vegetables, whole grains, legumes, nuts, and seeds, while also incorporating fish and seafood for protein and essential nutrients like omega-3 fatty acids.

Ingredients:

- Fish and Seafood: Salmon, trout, tuna, mackerel, shrimp, scallops, etc.

- Plant-Based Foods: Fruits, vegetables, whole grains, legumes, nuts, seeds.

- Dairy and Eggs: Milk, cheese, yogurt, eggs (optional, depending on individual preferences).

- Healthy Fats: Avocado, olive oil, nuts, seeds.

- Herbs and Spices: Basil, oregano, garlic, turmeric, ginger, etc.

Instructions/How to Prepare:

1. Base meals around plant-based foods such as fruits, vegetables, whole grains, legumes, nuts, and seeds.

2. Incorporate fish and seafood into meals as the primary source of protein.

3. Choose fatty fish like salmon, mackerel, and trout for their omega-3 fatty acids.

4. Include dairy products and eggs if desired and tolerated, as they provide additional protein and nutrients.

5. Use healthy fats like avocado, olive oil, nuts, and seeds for cooking and dressing.

6. Experiment with a variety of cooking methods, such as grilling, baking, steaming, and sautéing, to enhance flavor and texture.

7. Be mindful of portion sizes and aim for balanced meals that include a variety of food groups.

8. Opt for whole, minimally processed foods and limit intake of processed and refined foods.

9. Stay hydrated by drinking plenty of water throughout the day.

10. Consider supplementing with vitamin B12 and vitamin D if fish and seafood are the primary sources of these nutrients in the diet.

Asian Diet:

Definition:

The Asian diet refers to the traditional eating patterns of countries in the Asian continent, which vary greatly depending on the region and cultural influences. However, some common characteristics include a high consumption of plant-based foods such as fruits, vegetables, whole grains, legumes, and nuts; moderate intake of lean proteins such as fish, poultry, tofu, and eggs; and limited consumption of red meat and processed foods. The Asian diet is known for its emphasis on balance, variety, and moderation, as well as the inclusion of herbs, spices, and fermented foods for flavor and health benefits.

Ingredients:

- Rice: White rice, brown rice, jasmine rice, basmati rice, etc.

- Vegetables: Leafy greens, bok choy, broccoli, cabbage, carrots, onions, garlic, etc.

- Seafood: Fish, shrimp, crab, squid, mussels, etc.

- Poultry: Chicken, duck, turkey (in moderation).

- Tofu and Soy Products: Tofu, tempeh, edamame, soy milk, etc.

- Fruits: Mangoes, papayas, lychees, durian, bananas, etc.

- Nuts and Seeds: Peanuts, cashews, almonds, sesame seeds, etc.

- Herbs and Spices: Ginger, garlic, turmeric, coriander, cumin, chili peppers, etc.

- Fermented Foods: Kimchi, miso, soy sauce, fermented tofu, pickled vegetables, etc.

Instructions/How to Prepare:

1. Base meals around rice, noodles, or other staple grains, which serve as the foundation of many Asian dishes.

2. Include a variety of colorful vegetables in meals for added vitamins, minerals, and fiber.

3. Incorporate seafood, poultry, tofu, or soy products as sources of protein, aiming for a balance between plant-based and animal-based proteins.

4. Use herbs, spices, and aromatics like ginger, garlic, turmeric, and chili peppers to add flavor to dishes without relying on added fats or sodium.

5. Opt for cooking methods such as stir-frying, steaming, boiling, and grilling to retain nutrients and minimize added fats.

6. Include fermented foods like kimchi, miso, and soy sauce for their probiotic and digestive health benefits.

7. Enjoy fruits and nuts as snacks or dessert options, incorporating them into meals for added sweetness and crunch.

8. Be mindful of portion sizes and avoid overeating, focusing on listening to your body's hunger and fullness cues.

9. Stay hydrated by drinking plenty of water, green tea, or herbal teas throughout the day.

10. Embrace the cultural diversity and culinary traditions of Asian cuisine by exploring recipes and ingredients from different regions.

Traditional Indian Diet:

Definition:

The traditional Indian diet is rooted in centuries-old culinary traditions and cultural practices, with a focus on balance, variety, and Ayurvedic principles of holistic health and wellness. It emphasizes plant-based foods such as whole grains, lentils, vegetables, fruits, nuts, and seeds, while also incorporating dairy products, lean proteins, and spices for flavor and medicinal purposes. The Indian diet is known for its use of aromatic spices, herbs, and cooking techniques that enhance both taste and nutritional value.

Ingredients:

- Whole Grains: Basmati rice, brown rice, wheat, millet, barley, quinoa, etc.

- Lentils and Legumes: Red lentils, chickpeas, black beans, mung beans, pigeon peas, etc.

- Vegetables: Spinach, potatoes, cauliflower, eggplant, okra, tomatoes, etc.

- Dairy Products: Milk, yogurt, paneer (Indian cheese), ghee (clarified butter), etc.

- Spices and Herbs: Turmeric, cumin, coriander, cardamom, cinnamon, cloves, ginger, garlic, etc.

- Fruits: Mangoes, bananas, apples, papayas, oranges, guavas, etc.

- Nuts and Seeds: Almonds, cashews, pistachios, peanuts, sesame seeds, etc.

- Lean Proteins: Chicken, fish, eggs (in moderation), tofu (less traditional), etc.

Instructions/How to Prepare:

1. Base meals around whole grains, lentils, and vegetables, which form the foundation of many traditional Indian dishes.

2. Incorporate a variety of lentils and legumes into meals for plant-based protein, fiber, and essential nutrients.

3. Use a wide array of spices and herbs to add flavor to dishes, such as turmeric, cumin, coriander, and ginger, which also offer medicinal properties.

4. Include dairy products like yogurt, paneer, and ghee for added calcium, protein, and healthy fats.

5. Opt for cooking methods such as sautéing, simmering, and pressure cooking to retain nutrients and enhance flavors.

6. Enjoy fruits as snacks or desserts, incorporating them into meals for natural sweetness and additional nutrients.

7. Include nuts and seeds in dishes or as snacks for added texture, flavor, and healthy fats.

8. Be mindful of portion sizes and avoid overeating, focusing on balanced meals that include a variety of food groups.

9. Stay hydrated by drinking water, herbal teas, or buttermilk throughout the day.

10. Embrace the cultural heritage and culinary traditions of Indian cuisine by exploring regional recipes and cooking techniques.

Low-Calorie Diet:

Definition:

A low-calorie diet is characterized by reducing daily calorie intake to create a calorie deficit, which can lead to weight loss. The focus is on consuming nutrient-dense foods that are lower in calories but still provide essential nutrients, such as vitamins, minerals, and fiber. This diet typically involves portion control, meal planning, and making healthier food choices to achieve and maintain a healthy weight.

Ingredients:

- Lean Proteins: Skinless poultry, fish, seafood, tofu, tempeh, legumes.

- Non-Starchy Vegetables: Leafy greens, broccoli, cauliflower, bell peppers, zucchini, etc.

- Whole Grains (in moderation): Quinoa, brown rice, whole wheat bread, oats, barley.

- Fruits (in moderation): Berries, apples, oranges, bananas, melons, etc.

- Healthy Fats (in moderation): Avocado, nuts, seeds, olive oil.

- Low-Calorie Flavor Enhancers: Herbs, spices, vinegar, lemon juice, mustard, hot sauce.

Instructions/How to Prepare:

1. Calculate your daily calorie needs based on your age, gender, weight, height, and activity level.

2. Set a calorie goal that creates a calorie deficit for weight loss, typically 500 to 1000 calories less than your maintenance calories.

3. Plan meals that include lean proteins, non-starchy vegetables, whole grains (in moderation), fruits (in moderation), and healthy fats (in moderation).

4. Incorporate low-calorie flavor enhancers such as herbs, spices, vinegar, lemon juice, mustard, and hot sauce to add flavor without adding extra calories.

5. Be mindful of portion sizes and avoid oversized servings, using smaller plates and utensils if necessary.

6. Focus on filling half of your plate with non-starchy vegetables to add volume and fiber to meals while keeping calories low.

7. Choose lean protein sources like skinless poultry, fish, tofu, and legumes to help satisfy hunger and maintain muscle mass.

8. Include whole grains and fruits in moderation for added nutrients and fiber, but be cautious of portion sizes to manage calorie intake.

9. Incorporate healthy fats like avocado, nuts, seeds, and olive oil into meals to promote satiety and provide essential fatty acids.

10. Stay hydrated by drinking plenty of water throughout the day, as thirst can sometimes be mistaken for hunger.

Gluten-Free Diet:

Definition:

A gluten-free diet involves eliminating foods that contain gluten, a protein found in wheat, barley, rye, and their derivatives. This diet is essential for individuals with celiac disease, an autoimmune disorder triggered by gluten, as well as those with non-celiac gluten sensitivity or wheat allergy. The gluten-free diet focuses on naturally gluten-free foods and gluten-free alternatives to grains containing gluten.

Ingredients:

- Naturally Gluten-Free Foods: Fruits, vegetables, nuts, seeds, legumes, meats, fish, seafood, eggs, dairy products.

- Gluten-Free Grains and Flours: Rice, quinoa, corn, millet, buckwheat, sorghum, amaranth, teff, gluten-free oats, almond flour, coconut flour, chickpea flour, etc.

- Gluten-Free Condiments and Flavorings: Tamari (gluten-free soy sauce), mustard, vinegar, herbs, spices, etc.

- Gluten-Free Snacks and Treats: Popcorn, rice cakes, gluten-free crackers, gluten-free cookies, dark chocolate, etc.

Instructions/How to Prepare:

1. Educate yourself about sources of gluten and read food labels carefully to identify gluten-containing ingredients.

2. Base meals around naturally gluten-free foods such as fruits, vegetables, nuts, seeds, legumes, meats, fish, seafood, eggs, and dairy products.

3. Choose gluten-free grains and flours as alternatives to wheat, barley, and rye, including rice, quinoa, corn, millet, buckwheat, and gluten-free oats.

4. Use gluten-free condiments and flavorings like tamari (gluten-free soy sauce), mustard, vinegar, herbs, and spices to add flavor to meals.

5. Be cautious of cross-contamination by using separate cooking utensils, cutting boards, and kitchen equipment for gluten-free foods.

6. Explore gluten-free alternatives to favorite dishes and snacks, such as gluten-free pasta, bread, crackers, and baked goods.

7. Experiment with gluten-free cooking and baking techniques using alternative flours like almond flour, coconut flour, and chickpea flour.

8. Be aware of hidden sources of gluten in processed foods, sauces, dressings, and packaged snacks, and choose certified gluten-free products when possible.

9. Check with restaurants about their gluten-free options and food preparation practices when dining out.

10.   Consider working with a registered dietitian or healthcare professional knowledgeable about gluten-free diets to ensure nutritional adequacy and dietary compliance.

Anti-Inflammatory Diet:

Definition:

An anti-inflammatory diet focuses on reducing inflammation in the body by emphasizing foods that have been shown to have anti-inflammatory properties while limiting or avoiding those that may contribute to inflammation. Chronic inflammation is associated with various health conditions, including heart disease, diabetes, arthritis, and certain cancers. The anti-inflammatory diet typically includes a variety of whole, nutrient-rich foods such as fruits, vegetables, whole grains, healthy fats, and lean proteins, while minimizing processed foods, refined sugars, and unhealthy fats.

Ingredients:

- Fruits: Berries, cherries, oranges, pineapple, papaya, etc.

- Vegetables: Leafy greens, broccoli, Brussels sprouts, cauliflower, sweet potatoes, etc.

- Whole Grains: Quinoa, brown rice, oats, barley, bulgur, whole wheat pasta.

- Healthy Fats: Avocado, olive oil, nuts, seeds, fatty fish (salmon, mackerel, sardines).

- Lean Proteins: Skinless poultry, fish, seafood, tofu, tempeh, legumes, beans.

- Herbs and Spices: Turmeric, ginger, garlic, cinnamon, cumin, basil, oregano, etc.

Instructions/How to Prepare:

1. Base meals around whole, nutrient-rich foods such as fruits, vegetables, whole grains, healthy fats, and lean proteins.

2. Incorporate a variety of colorful fruits and vegetables into meals and snacks for their antioxidants and anti-inflammatory compounds.

3. Choose whole grains like quinoa, brown rice, and oats over refined grains for added fiber and nutrients.

4. Include healthy fats like avocado, olive oil, nuts, and seeds in moderation to reduce inflammation and support overall health.

5. Opt for lean protein sources such as fish, poultry, tofu, and legumes, which contain anti-inflammatory properties.

6. Flavor dishes with herbs and spices like turmeric, ginger, garlic, cinnamon, and cumin, which have been shown to have anti-inflammatory effects.

7. Minimize consumption of processed foods, refined sugars, and unhealthy fats, which can contribute to inflammation.

8. Be mindful of portion sizes and avoid overeating, focusing on listening to your body's hunger and fullness cues.

9. Stay hydrated by drinking plenty of water throughout the day, as dehydration can exacerbate inflammation.

10. Aim for a balanced diet that includes a variety of nutrient-dense foods while reducing sources of inflammation, and consider consulting with a healthcare

professional or registered dietitian for personalized guidance and support.

Specific Carbohydrate Diet (SCD):

Definition:

The Specific Carbohydrate Diet (SCD) is a dietary regimen designed to manage certain digestive disorders, particularly inflammatory bowel diseases (IBD) such as Crohn's disease, ulcerative colitis, and celiac disease. It aims to reduce inflammation and promote healing of the gastrointestinal tract by restricting certain carbohydrates that are thought to exacerbate symptoms. The diet focuses on consuming easily digestible, nutrient-rich foods that are low in carbohydrates and free of complex sugars and starches.

Ingredients:

- Fresh Fruits: Apples, bananas, berries, melons, etc.

- Non-Starchy Vegetables: Leafy greens, carrots, cucumbers, bell peppers, squash, etc.

- Lean Proteins: Chicken, turkey, fish, eggs, tofu, tempeh, and certain cuts of beef or pork.

- Healthy Fats: Olive oil, coconut oil, avocados, nuts, seeds.

- Fermented Foods (in moderation): Yogurt, kefir, sauerkraut, kimchi.

- Certain Legumes and Beans (in limited amounts): Lentils, black beans, navy beans.

- Homemade Broths and Soups: Chicken broth, bone broth, vegetable soup.

- Natural Sweeteners (in moderation): Honey, maple syrup.

Instructions/How to Prepare:

1. Eliminate complex carbohydrates such as grains, processed foods, and sugars from the diet.

2. Base meals around fresh fruits, non-starchy vegetables, lean proteins, and healthy fats.

3. Choose easily digestible proteins such as poultry, fish, eggs, tofu, and tempeh.

4. Incorporate healthy fats like olive oil, coconut oil, avocados, nuts, and seeds into meals for satiety and energy.

5. Include fermented foods like yogurt, kefir, sauerkraut, and kimchi in moderation to support gut health and digestion.

6. Experiment with homemade broths and soups made from scratch using nutrient-rich ingredients.

7. Be cautious with certain legumes and beans, as they may cause digestive discomfort in some individuals.

8. Use natural sweeteners like honey and maple syrup sparingly, as they are allowed in moderation on the SCD.

9. Avoid processed foods, artificial additives, and preservatives, opting for whole, unprocessed foods whenever possible.

10. Monitor symptoms and adjust the diet as needed to manage digestive issues and promote overall well-being, and consider consulting with a healthcare professional or registered dietitian for personalized guidance and support.

Zone Diet:

Definition:

The Zone Diet is a low-glycemic, moderate-protein, and moderate-fat eating plan designed to optimize hormone levels, promote weight loss, and improve overall health and performance. It aims to balance macronutrients in a specific ratio to control inflammation, stabilize blood sugar levels, and enhance metabolic function. The diet emphasizes portion control and consuming meals that are rich in protein, low in carbohydrates, and include healthy fats to maintain a state of "the zone," where the body efficiently burns fat for fuel.

Ingredients:

- Lean Proteins: Skinless poultry, fish, seafood, tofu, tempeh, lean cuts of beef or pork.

- Non-Starchy Vegetables: Leafy greens, broccoli, cauliflower, bell peppers, zucchini, spinach, etc.

- Healthy Fats: Olive oil, avocado, nuts, seeds, fatty fish (salmon, mackerel, sardines).

- Low-Glycemic Carbohydrates (in moderation): Berries, apples, oranges, quinoa, brown rice, sweet potatoes.

- Some Dairy Products (in moderation): Greek yogurt, cottage cheese, low-fat cheese.

Instructions/How to Prepare:

1. Divide meals into specific portions of protein, carbohydrates, and fats to achieve the desired macronutrient ratio (40% carbohydrates, 30% protein, 30% fat).

2. Base meals around lean proteins such as poultry, fish, seafood, tofu, and tempeh, aiming for a portion size that fits in the palm of your hand.

3. Include plenty of non-starchy vegetables like leafy greens, broccoli, cauliflower, and bell peppers to bulk up meals and add fiber and nutrients.

4. Incorporate healthy fats like olive oil, avocado, nuts, and seeds into meals for satiety and to help balance blood sugar levels.

5. Choose low-glycemic carbohydrates such as berries, apples, oranges, quinoa, brown rice, and sweet potatoes to minimize spikes in blood sugar.

6. Be mindful of portion sizes and avoid overeating, focusing on balanced meals that include a variety of food groups.

7. Include some dairy products like Greek yogurt, cottage cheese, and low-fat cheese in moderation for additional protein and calcium.

8. Plan meals and snacks ahead of time to ensure they fit within the macronutrient ratio and support your nutritional goals.

9. Stay hydrated by drinking plenty of water throughout the day to support metabolic function and overall health.

10. Monitor progress and adjust portion sizes and food choices as needed to achieve and maintain the desired balance of macronutrients, and consider consulting with a healthcare professional or registered dietitian for personalized guidance and support.

Engine 2 Diet:

Definition:

The Engine 2 Diet, developed by firefighter Rip Esselstyn, is a plant-based eating plan designed to promote heart health, weight loss, and overall well-being. It emphasizes whole, nutrient-dense, plant-based foods while minimizing or eliminating animal products, oils, processed foods, and added sugars. The diet is inspired by the idea that eating "like a firefighter" – with a focus on whole plant foods – can prevent and even reverse chronic diseases such as heart disease, diabetes, and obesity.

Ingredients:

- Whole Grains: Brown rice, quinoa, oats, barley, whole wheat pasta, whole grain bread.

- Beans and Legumes: Black beans, lentils, chickpeas, kidney beans, edamame, tofu.

- Fruits: Berries, apples, oranges, bananas, mangoes, melons, etc.

- Vegetables: Leafy greens, broccoli, cauliflower, bell peppers, carrots, onions, etc.

- Nuts and Seeds (in moderation): Almonds, walnuts, chia seeds, flaxseeds, hemp seeds, etc.

- Herbs and Spices: Basil, oregano, garlic, ginger, turmeric, cumin, etc.

Instructions/How to Prepare:

1. Base meals around whole, plant-based foods such as whole grains, beans, legumes, fruits, and vegetables.

2. Include a variety of colorful fruits and vegetables in meals and snacks for their vitamins, minerals, and antioxidants.

3. Choose whole grains like brown rice, quinoa, oats, and barley for fiber and nutrients.

4. Incorporate beans and legumes into meals for plant-based protein, fiber, and essential nutrients.

5. Limit or eliminate processed foods, oils, added sugars, and animal products from the diet.

6. Use nuts and seeds sparingly for added texture and flavor, as they are high in calories.

7. Flavor dishes with herbs and spices instead of salt or added fats to enhance taste without extra calories.

8. Experiment with plant-based cooking techniques such as steaming, sautéing, roasting, and grilling to bring out natural flavors.

9. Be mindful of portion sizes and avoid overeating, focusing on balanced meals that include a variety of food groups.

10. Stay hydrated by drinking plenty of water throughout the day, and consider incorporating regular physical activity to complement dietary changes.

Dr. Bernstein's Diabetes Diet:

Definition:

Dr. Richard K. Bernstein's Diabetes Diet is a low-carbohydrate eating plan specifically designed to manage blood sugar levels and improve health outcomes for individuals with diabetes, particularly type 1 diabetes. It emphasizes controlling carbohydrate intake to prevent spikes in blood sugar, achieve stable glucose levels, and reduce the need for insulin medication. The diet consists of whole, nutrient-dense foods that are low in carbohydrates but rich in protein, healthy fats, fiber, vitamins, and minerals.

Ingredients:

- Non-Starchy Vegetables: Leafy greens, broccoli, cauliflower, bell peppers, zucchini, spinach, etc.

- Lean Proteins: Chicken, turkey, fish, seafood, eggs, tofu, tempeh, lean cuts of beef or pork.

- Healthy Fats: Olive oil, avocado, nuts, seeds, fatty fish (salmon, mackerel, sardines).

- Low-Glycemic Carbohydrates (in moderation): Berries, apples, oranges, quinoa, brown rice, sweet potatoes.

- Some Dairy Products (in moderation): Greek yogurt, cottage cheese, low-fat cheese.

Instructions/How to Prepare:

1. Limit carbohydrate intake to a specific amount per meal, typically 15 grams or less for breakfast and 30 grams or less for lunch and dinner.

2. Base meals around non-starchy vegetables, which are low in carbohydrates and high in fiber, vitamins, and minerals.

3. Include lean proteins such as poultry, fish, seafood, eggs, tofu, and tempeh in each meal to help stabilize blood sugar levels and promote satiety.

4. Incorporate healthy fats like olive oil, avocado, nuts, and seeds into meals for sustained energy and to slow the absorption of carbohydrates.

5. Choose low-glycemic carbohydrates like berries, apples, oranges, quinoa, brown rice, and sweet potatoes in moderation to minimize spikes in blood sugar.

6. Be cautious with portion sizes and avoid overeating, especially with carbohydrate-rich foods.

7. Monitor blood sugar levels regularly and adjust carbohydrate intake, insulin medication, and dietary choices as needed to maintain stable glucose levels.

8. Plan meals and snacks ahead of time to ensure they fit within the carbohydrate limits and support blood sugar control.

9. Stay hydrated by drinking plenty of water throughout the day, and consider incorporating regular physical activity to improve insulin sensitivity and overall health.

10. Work closely with a healthcare professional or registered dietitian experienced in diabetes management to develop a personalized meal plan and monitor progress over time.

Raw Food Diet:

Definition:

The raw food diet is based on the belief that consuming foods in their natural, uncooked state provides maximum nutritional benefits and enzymes that are destroyed during cooking. This diet typically includes raw fruits, vegetables, nuts, seeds, sprouted grains, and legumes, as well as some raw or minimally processed dairy products, eggs, fish, and meat. The raw food diet is high in vitamins, minerals, fiber, and antioxidants, and proponents believe it can lead to improved digestion, increased energy, weight loss, and reduced risk of chronic diseases.

Ingredients:

- Raw Fruits: Berries, apples, oranges, bananas, mangoes, etc.

- Raw Vegetables: Leafy greens, carrots, cucumbers, bell peppers, tomatoes, etc.

- Nuts and Seeds: Almonds, walnuts, cashews, sunflower seeds, chia seeds, flaxseeds, etc.

- Sprouted Grains and Legumes: Sprouted quinoa, lentils, chickpeas, mung beans, etc.

- Raw Dairy and Eggs (if consumed): Raw milk, cheese, yogurt, eggs (in moderation).

- Raw or Minimally Processed Meat and Fish (if consumed): Sashimi, ceviche, carpaccio, etc.

- Cold-Pressed Oils: Olive oil, coconut oil, flaxseed oil, etc.

Instructions/How to Prepare:

1. Base meals around raw fruits, vegetables, nuts, seeds, sprouted grains, and legumes.

2. Incorporate a variety of colorful fruits and vegetables into meals and snacks for their vitamins, minerals, and antioxidants.

3. Include nuts and seeds for healthy fats, protein, and fiber, using them in salads, smoothies, or raw energy bars.

4. Experiment with sprouted grains and legumes, which are easier to digest and may have increased nutrient bioavailability.

5. Be cautious with raw dairy and eggs, choosing high-quality, pasteurized options to reduce the risk of foodborne illness.

6. If consuming raw meat or fish, ensure it is fresh, high-quality, and properly handled to minimize the risk of foodborne pathogens.

7. Use cold-pressed oils like olive oil, coconut oil, and flaxseed oil for dressing salads or adding flavor to dishes.

8. Be creative with food preparation techniques such as blending, juicing, dehydrating, and marinating to enhance flavor and texture.

9. Be mindful of food safety practices when handling raw foods, including washing produce thoroughly and storing perishable items properly.

10. Listen to your body and adjust the raw food diet to meet your individual nutritional needs, and consider consulting with a healthcare professional or registered dietitian for personalized guidance and support.

Nordic Diet:

Definition:

The Nordic diet is a traditional eating pattern inspired by the cuisines of countries in the Nordic region, such as Denmark, Finland, Iceland, Norway, and Sweden. It emphasizes seasonal, locally sourced foods that are typical of the region, including fish, seafood, whole grains, berries, root vegetables, legumes, and rapeseed oil. The diet is characterized by its high fiber, low glycemic index, and focus on quality ingredients.

Ingredients:

- Fish and Seafood: Salmon, herring, mackerel, cod, trout, shrimp, etc.

- Whole Grains: Rye bread, barley, oats, quinoa, whole grain pasta.

- Berries: Blueberries, lingonberries, raspberries, cloudberries, etc.

- Vegetables: Root vegetables (e.g., carrots, potatoes, beets), leafy greens, cabbage, onions, etc.

- Legumes: Beans, lentils, peas.

- Rapeseed Oil: Used for cooking and dressing.

- Dairy: Milk, cheese, yogurt (in moderation).

- Herbs and Spices: Dill, parsley, thyme, juniper berries, etc.

Instructions/How to Prepare:

1. Base meals around seasonal, locally sourced foods typical of the Nordic region.

2. Include fish and seafood as the primary sources of protein, aiming for 2-3 servings per week.

3. Incorporate whole grains such as rye bread, barley, oats, and quinoa into meals for fiber and nutrients.

4. Enjoy a variety of berries, which are rich in antioxidants and vitamins.

5. Include plenty of vegetables, particularly root vegetables, leafy greens, and cabbage.

6. Incorporate legumes like beans, lentils, and peas into soups, stews, and salads for plant-based protein and fiber.

7. Use rapeseed oil for cooking and dressing, as it's a traditional oil in Nordic cuisine and rich in omega-3 fatty acids.

8. Include dairy products like milk, cheese, and yogurt in moderation, opting for low-fat or fermented varieties.

9. Flavor dishes with traditional Nordic herbs and spices like dill, parsley, thyme, and juniper berries.

10. Be mindful of portion sizes and aim for balanced meals that include a variety of food groups, focusing on quality ingredients and seasonal produce.

Here's a 31-day meal plan based on recipes from a budget-friendly diabetic cookbook for those newly diagnosed:

CHAPTER 12

31 DAY MEAL PLAN

Week 1:

Day 1:

- Breakfast: Scrambled eggs with spinach and tomatoes.

- Lunch: Turkey and cheese sandwich on whole grain bread with a side salad.

- Dinner: Baked chicken breast with roasted vegetables (carrots, broccoli, and cauliflower).

Day 2:

- Breakfast: Oatmeal with sliced strawberries and a sprinkle of cinnamon.

- Lunch: Tuna salad with mixed greens and cucumbers.

- Dinner: Lentil soup with a side of whole grain bread.

Day 3:

- Breakfast: Greek yogurt with sliced bananas and a drizzle of honey.

- Lunch: Vegetable stir-fry with tofu and brown rice.

- Dinner: Baked fish (like tilapia or cod) with steamed green beans.

Day 4:

- Breakfast: Whole grain toast with avocado and poached eggs.
- Lunch: Quinoa salad with diced bell peppers, cucumber, and feta cheese.
- Dinner: Turkey meatballs in marinara sauce with zucchini noodles.

Day 5:

- Breakfast: Smoothie with spinach, berries, almond milk, and protein powder.
- Lunch: Chicken and vegetable kebabs with a side of Greek salad.
- Dinner: Stir-fried tofu with mixed vegetables and brown rice.

Week 2:

Day 6:

- Breakfast: Cottage cheese with sliced peaches and a sprinkle of cinnamon.
- Lunch: Black bean and corn salad with avocado and lime dressing.
- Dinner: Spaghetti squash with marinara sauce and a side of roasted asparagus.

Day 7:

- Breakfast: Whole grain waffles with Greek yogurt and mixed berries.

- Lunch: Turkey and cheese roll-ups with lettuce and mustard.

- Dinner: Chili made with lean ground turkey, beans, and tomatoes.

Day 8:

- Breakfast: Egg muffins with spinach, mushrooms, and cheese.

- Lunch: Caprese salad with sliced tomatoes, mozzarella, and basil.

- Dinner: Baked pork chops with roasted sweet potatoes.

Day 9:

- Breakfast: Smoothie bowl with spinach, banana, almond milk, and granola.

- Lunch: Chickpea salad with cucumber, tomatoes, and feta cheese.

- Dinner: Grilled shrimp with quinoa and steamed broccoli.

Day 10:

- Breakfast: Whole grain toast with almond butter and sliced apples.

- Lunch: Lentil soup with a side of mixed greens.

- Dinner: Baked chicken thighs with roasted Brussels sprouts.

Week 3:

Day 11:

- Breakfast: Yogurt parfait with granola and mixed berries.

- Lunch: Turkey lettuce wraps with sliced bell peppers.

- Dinner: Baked salmon with roasted carrots.

Day 12:

- Breakfast: Whole grain cereal with low-fat milk and sliced bananas.

- Lunch: Spinach and feta stuffed chicken breast.

- Dinner: Stir-fried beef with broccoli and brown rice.

Day 13:

- Breakfast: Peanut butter and banana sandwich on whole grain bread.

- Lunch: Quinoa and black bean stuffed peppers.

- Dinner: Grilled steak with sautéed spinach.

Day 14:

- Breakfast: Overnight oats with almond milk, chia seeds, and berries.
- Lunch: Chicken Caesar salad with homemade dressing.
- Dinner: Baked cod with roasted cauliflower.

Day 15:

- Breakfast: Scrambled eggs with diced bell peppers and onions.
- Lunch: Turkey and vegetable stir-fry with brown rice.
- Dinner: Grilled tofu with grilled vegetables.

Week 4:

Day 16:

- Breakfast: Whole grain pancakes with Greek yogurt and sliced strawberries.
- Lunch: Egg salad with mixed greens and cherry tomatoes.
- Dinner: Baked tilapia with quinoa and steamed green beans.

Day 17:

- Breakfast: Greek yogurt with sliced peaches and a sprinkle of cinnamon.

- Lunch: Veggie wrap with hummus, lettuce, and tomato.

- Dinner: Turkey chili with a side of whole grain bread.

Day 18:

- Breakfast: Smoothie with spinach, mango, almond milk, and protein powder.

- Lunch: Tomato and mozzarella salad with balsamic vinaigrette.

- Dinner: Baked chicken breast with roasted vegetables (carrots, broccoli, and cauliflower).

Day 19:

- Breakfast: Whole grain toast with avocado and poached eggs.

- Lunch: Lentil salad with cucumber, tomatoes, and olives.

- Dinner: Stir-fried tofu with mixed vegetables and brown rice.

Day 20:

- Breakfast: Cottage cheese with sliced bananas and a sprinkle of cinnamon.

- Lunch: Turkey and cheese sandwich on whole grain bread with a side salad.

- Dinner: Baked fish (like tilapia or cod) with steamed green beans.

Week 5:

Day 21:

- Breakfast: Oatmeal with sliced strawberries and a sprinkle of cinnamon.

- Lunch: Tuna salad with mixed greens and cucumbers.

- Dinner: Turkey meatballs in marinara sauce with zucchini noodles.

Day 22:

- Breakfast: Greek yogurt with mixed berries and a drizzle of honey.

- Lunch: Vegetable stir-fry with tofu and brown rice.

- Dinner: Baked pork chops with roasted sweet potatoes.

Day 23:

- Breakfast: Whole grain waffles with Greek yogurt and mixed berries.

- Lunch: Chicken and vegetable kebabs with a side of Greek salad.

- Dinner: Stir-fried tofu with mixed vegetables and brown rice.

Day 24:

- Breakfast: Cottage cheese with sliced peaches and a sprinkle of cinnamon.

- Lunch: Black bean and corn salad with avocado and lime dressing.

- Dinner: Spaghetti squash with marinara sauce and a side of roasted asparagus.

Day 25:

- Breakfast: Smoothie with spinach, berries, almond milk, and protein powder.

- Lunch: Turkey and cheese roll-ups with lettuce and mustard.

- Dinner: Chili made with lean ground turkey, beans, and tomatoes.

Week 6:

Day 26:

- Breakfast: Egg muffins with spinach, mushrooms, and cheese.

- Lunch: Caprese salad with sliced tomatoes, mozzarella, and basil.

- Dinner: Baked pork chops with roasted sweet potatoes.

Day 27:

- Breakfast: Smoothie bowl with spinach, banana, almond milk, and granola.
- Lunch: Chickpea salad with cucumber, tomatoes, and feta cheese.
- Dinner: Grilled shrimp with quinoa and steamed broccoli.

Day 28:

- Breakfast: Whole grain toast with almond butter and sliced apples.
- Lunch: Lentil soup with a side of mixed greens.
- Dinner: Baked chicken thighs with roasted Brussels sprouts.

Day 29:

- Breakfast: Yogurt parfait with granola and mixed berries.
- Lunch: Turkey lettuce wraps with sliced bell peppers.
- Dinner: Baked salmon with roasted carrots.

Day 30:

- Breakfast: Whole grain cereal with low-fat milk and sliced bananas.
- Lunch: Spinach and feta stuffed chicken breast.

- Dinner: Stir-fried beef with broccoli and brown rice.

Day 31:

- Breakfast: Peanut butter and banana sandwich on whole grain bread.

- Lunch: Quinoa and black bean stuffed peppers.

- Dinner: Grilled steak with sautéed spinach.

THE END